# Cytotec

# and

# Mifepristone

# User Guide Book

Understanding the mechanism of action, containdications, monitoring symptoms, follow up care for Safe and Effective Use for medical Abortion

Dr. Jane Miles

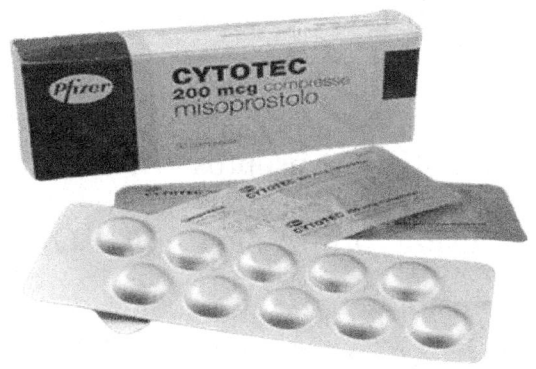

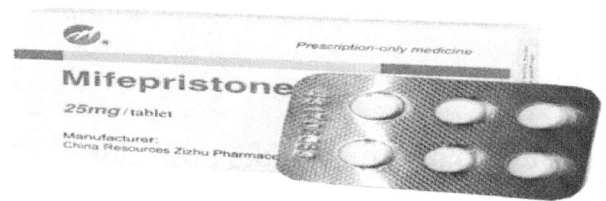

3 | cytotec and mifepristone manual book

# TABLE OF CONTENTS

# Introduction

## What is Cytotec (Misoprostol)?

**Cytotec**

(Misoprostol) is a medication used to prevent and treat stomach ulcers, particularly in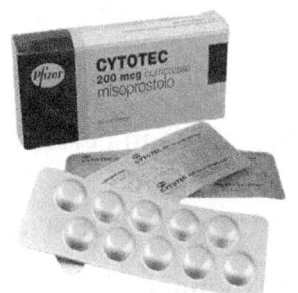
patients taking nonsteroidal anti-inflammatory drugs (NSAIDs) such as aspirin and ibuprofen. It works by reducing stomach acid and protecting the stomach lining from irritation. Misoprostol is a synthetic form of prostaglandin, a substance that naturally occurs in the body and helps protect the stomach lining.

In addition to its use for ulcer prevention, Cytotec is sometimes prescribed for other medical purposes, including:

**Inducing Labor:** Cytotec can be used to soften the cervix and stimulate uterine contractions in certain situations.

**Managing Miscarriage:** It is also used to help manage incomplete miscarriages by encouraging the expulsion of pregnancy tissue.

**Medical Abortion:** Misoprostol is commonly combined with another medication, mifepristone, to terminate early pregnancies.

# Mechanism of Action of Cytotec (Misoprostol)

**Cytotec** primarily works by mimicking the hormone prostaglandin E2. Prostaglandins are naturally occurring substances that play a crucial role in various bodily functions, including uterine contractions.

When Cytotec is used to induce labor or facilitate medical abortions, it works in the following ways:

**Uterine Contractions**: Cytotec stimulates the uterus to contract, which can help to dilate the cervix and expel the fetus or uterine contents.

**Cervical Softening**: By mimicking prostaglandins, Cytotec can soften the cervix, making it more pliable and easier for the fetus to pass through.

**Blood Vessel Contraction**: Cytotec can also cause blood vessels in the uterus to contract, reducing blood flow and helping to control bleeding.

A medical abortion is a non-surgical procedure used to terminate a pregnancy in the early stages. It typically involves the use of medications to induce a miscarriage.

**Commonly used medications:**

**Misoprostol:** This medication is often used in combination with mifepristone to induce a medical abortion.

**Mifepristone:** This medication blocks the action of progesterone, a hormone necessary for maintaining pregnancy.

**How it works:**

**Mifepristone:** This medication is taken orally and blocks the action of progesterone, causing the uterine lining to break down.

**Misoprostol:** This medication is taken orally or vaginally a few days after mifepristone. It causes the uterus to contract, expelling the pregnancy tissue.

**Important notes:**

Medical abortions are typically safe and effective when performed under the guidance of a healthcare professional.

The effectiveness of medical abortions depends on factors such as the gestational age and the individual's health.

It's crucial to follow the instructions provided by your healthcare provider and to be aware of potential side effects and complications.

# Section 2: Before Use

## When to use Cytotec

Cytotec is typically used in the early stages of pregnancy to induce a medical abortion. The effectiveness of Cytotec in inducing a medical abortion decreases as the pregnancy progresses.

Generally, Cytotec is most effective when used:

**Within the first 10 weeks of pregnancy:** This is the optimal time frame for using Cytotec for a medical abortion.

**Up to 12 weeks of pregnancy**: In some cases, Cytotec may be effective up to 12 weeks of pregnancy, but the success rate may be lower.

Risks and side effects While Cytotec is generally safe when used as directed by a healthcare professional, there are potential risks and side effects associated with its use.

**Common side effects of Cytotec may include:**

Abdominal cramping and pain

Bleeding (which can be heavy)

Nausea and vomiting

Diarrhea

Fever

Chills

Fatigue

Headache

**More serious side effects are less common but can occur. These may include:**

Incomplete abortion (retained tissue)

Infection

Excessive bleeding

Allergic reactions

**If you experience any of these or other concerning symptoms while using Cytotec, it's crucial to seek immediate medical attention.**

## Contraindications

Cytotec should not be used in certain circumstances. These contraindications include:

**Pregnancy beyond 12 weeks:** Cytotec is generally not effective or safe for use after 12 weeks of pregnancy.

**Ectopic pregnancy:** If you have an ectopic pregnancy (a pregnancy that implants outside the uterus), Cytotec should not be used.

**Severe anemia:** Women with severe anemia may be at increased risk of complications from Cytotec use.

**Chronic kidney or liver disease:** These conditions can affect how your body processes Cytotec.

**History of pelvic inflammatory disease (PID):** PID can increase the risk of infection after using Cytotec.

**Certain medications:** Cytotec may interact with other medications you are taking.

## Preparing for the procedure

Before using Cytotec, it's essential to follow the instructions provided by your healthcare provider. This may involve:

Confirming your pregnancy: Your healthcare provider will likely perform a pregnancy test to confirm the gestational age and viability of the pregnancy.

Understanding the risks and benefits: You should discuss the potential risks and benefits of using Cytotec with your healthcare provider.

Preparing your home environment: Create a comfortable and private space where you can rest after taking Cytotec.

Gathering necessary supplies: You may need to gather supplies such as pads, pain relievers, and a thermometer.

# Section 3: The Procedure

## How to take Cytotec

Typical Cytotec dosages for medical abortion:

**Early pregnancy (up to 12 weeks):**

Oral: 200 micrograms (mcg) taken every 3 hours, for a total of 800 mcg over 24 hours.

Vaginal: 800 mcg inserted vaginally, followed by 400 mcg 24 hours later.

**Later pregnancy (12-14 weeks):**

Oral: Higher dosages may be recommended, but the specific dosage will depend on your healthcare provider's instructions.

## What to expect during the procedure

When using Cytotec for a medical abortion, you can expect to experience some symptoms. These may include:

**Cramping and pain:** You may experience abdominal cramping and pain similar to menstrual cramps.

**Bleeding:** Bleeding can vary in intensity and may last for several days.

**Nausea and vomiting:** Some women may experience nausea or vomiting.

**Chills and fever:** You may also experience chills or a low-grade fever.

The procedure typically takes place at home or in a private setting. You may be advised to rest and avoid strenuous activity during the procedure.

It's important to note that the experience can vary from person to person. Some women may experience more intense symptoms than others.

If you experience any severe or unusual symptoms, such as excessive bleeding, severe pain, or signs of infection, it's crucial to seek immediate medical attention.

## Possible complications

While Cytotec is generally safe when used under the guidance of a healthcare professional, there are potential complications associated with its use. These can include:

**Incomplete abortion:** This occurs when some of the pregnancy tissue remains in the uterus. If not treated, it can lead to infection or bleeding.

**Infection:** There is a risk of infection, especially if the abortion is not complete.

**Excessive bleeding:** While some bleeding is normal after a medical abortion, excessive bleeding can be a concern.

**Hemorrhage:** In rare cases, severe bleeding (hemorrhage) can occur.

**Allergic reactions:** Some people may experience allergic reactions to Cytotec.

**Emotional distress:** The experience of a medical abortion can be emotionally challenging for some women.

**If you experience any of these or other concerning symptoms while using Cytotec, it's crucial to seek immediate medical attention.**

# Section 4: Aftercare

## Monitoring Symptoms

After using Cytotec, it's important to monitor your symptoms closely. This includes:

**Bleeding:** Keep track of the amount and color of your bleeding. If you experience excessive bleeding or bleeding that lasts for more than a week, contact your healthcare provider.

**Pain:** Note any abdominal pain or cramping you experience. If the pain is severe or persistent, contact your healthcare provider.

**Fever:** Monitor your temperature for any signs of fever. A fever could indicate an infection.

**Other symptoms:** Pay attention to any other symptoms you may experience, such as nausea, vomiting, or dizziness.

## Follow-up Care

Your healthcare provider will likely schedule a follow-up appointment to check on your progress and ensure that the abortion was complete. During this appointment, they may perform a physical exam and possibly an ultrasound to confirm that the uterus is empty.

It's important to attend this follow-up appointment, even if you feel fine. Your healthcare provider can address any concerns you may have and provide guidance on ongoing care.

## Disposal of Unused Medication

**Never flush unused medication down the toilet.** This can contaminate the water supply. Instead, dispose of unused Cytotec according to the instructions provided by your healthcare provider or local regulations. This may involve returning the medication to a pharmacy for proper disposal.

# Section 5: Frequently Asked Questions

## Common Questions About Cytotec

**1. Is Cytotec safe?**

Cytotec is generally safe when used under the guidance of a healthcare professional. However, like any medication, it carries potential risks and side effects. It's crucial to weigh the risks and benefits with your healthcare provider.

**2. How effective is Cytotec for medical abortions?**

The effectiveness of Cytotec for medical abortions depends on factors such as the gestational age and the individual's health.

Generally, it's most effective in the early stages of pregnancy.

## 3. Can I use Cytotec at home?

While it's possible to use Cytotec at home, it's strongly recommended to do so under the supervision of a healthcare professional. They can provide guidance, monitor your progress, and address any complications that may arise.

## 4. Is it painful to use Cytotec?

You may experience cramping and pain after using Cytotec, similar to menstrual cramps. The intensity of pain can vary from person to person.

## 5. How long does it take for Cytotec to work?

The time it takes for Cytotec to work can vary. You may start to experience symptoms within a few hours of taking the medication. However, it may take several days for the abortion to be complete.

## 6. Can I get pregnant again after using Cytotec?

Yes, you can get pregnant again after using Cytotec. It's important to use contraception to prevent pregnancy if you are sexually active.

## 7. Can I use Cytotec to induce labor?

Cytotec may be used to induce labor in certain circumstances, but this should only be done under the guidance of a healthcare professional.

## 8. What if I have a reaction to Cytotec?

If you experience any severe or unusual symptoms while using Cytotec, such as excessive bleeding, severe pain, or signs of infection, it's crucial to seek immediate medical attention.

**9. Is it possible to have an incomplete abortion after using Cytotec?**

Yes, there is a risk of incomplete abortion. If you experience persistent bleeding or other symptoms after using Cytotec, it's important to follow up with your healthcare provider.

**10. Can I use Cytotec if I have an ectopic pregnancy?**

No, Cytotec should not be used if you have an ectopic pregnancy. Ectopic pregnancies can be dangerous and require immediate medical attention.

# CHAPTER 2

# MIFEPRISTONE

**Mifepristone** is a medication that has become a significant tool in the field of reproductive health,

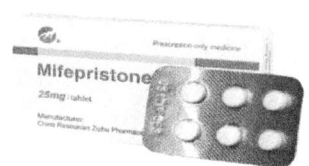

particularly in the context of medical abortion. Originally developed for the purpose of terminating early pregnancies, mifepristone works by blocking the hormone progesterone, which is essential for maintaining a pregnancy. When used in combination with misoprostol, mifepristone has proven to be a highly effective method for safely terminating a pregnancy without the need for surgical intervention.

## What is Mifepristone?

Mifepristone, also known by its brand name RU-486, is a synthetic steroid that is used primarily as a medication to induce medical abortion in the early stages of pregnancy. It is typically prescribed up to 10 weeks of gestation. By inhibiting the action of progesterone, a hormone critical to sustaining the uterine lining and supporting embryo implantation, mifepristone prepares the body for the expulsion of the pregnancy.

In addition to its use in abortion, mifepristone has other medical applications, including treating Cushing's syndrome and managing certain conditions related to the uterus, such as fibroids.

## How Does Mifepristone Work?

**Mifepristone** works by blocking the hormone progesterone, which is crucial for maintaining a pregnancy. Progesterone helps thicken the lining of the uterus, creating a supportive environment for the developing embryo. When mifepristone is taken, it effectively inhibits this process, causing the uterine lining to break down, making it unable to support the pregnancy. This leads to the detachment of the pregnancy from the uterine wall.

After taking mifepristone, misoprostol is typically administered 24 to 48 hours later to induce uterine contractions, facilitating the expulsion of the pregnancy tissue. The combination of these two medications results in a complete abortion in most cases, making it a non-invasive alternative to surgical procedures.

## Medical Abortion: A Brief Overview

Medical abortion is a non-surgical method of terminating an early pregnancy using medication rather than instruments or anesthesia. The most common regimen involves two drugs: mifepristone and misoprostol. Mifepristone is taken first to block progesterone and begin the process of terminating the pregnancy. Misoprostol, which is taken shortly after, induces contractions of the uterus, helping the body expel the pregnancy tissue.

Medical abortion is considered safe and effective when performed within the first 10 weeks of pregnancy. It offers an option for those seeking a more private and less invasive alternative to surgical abortion. The process usually takes a few days, and while it can involve cramping and bleeding similar to a heavy menstrual period, it generally does not require hospitalization.

Medical abortion is widely used around the world and is often preferred due to its convenience and effectiveness. However, it is essential to have medical supervision to ensure safety and to handle any potential complications that may arise.

# Section 2: Before Use

Understanding how and when to use mifepristone, along with its potential risks and necessary preparations, is crucial for ensuring both safety and effectiveness in the process of medical abortion. This section will explore when mifepristone is appropriate, its associated risks, contraindications, and how to prepare for the procedure.

## When to Use Mifepristone

Mifepristone is generally prescribed for medical abortions within the first 10 weeks of pregnancy, measured from the first day of the last menstrual period (LMP). This period is considered ideal because the pregnancy is still early, and the combination of mifepristone and misoprostol is most effective and least likely to result in complications.

Aside from its use in medical abortion, mifepristone may also be used in some cases to manage miscarriages, treat certain uterine conditions, or in the treatment of Cushing's syndrome. However, when prescribed for abortion, it is critical that the gestational age is accurately assessed, usually through an ultrasound, to ensure that the medication is being used safely within the recommended timeframe.

## Risks and Side Effects

Like all medications, mifepristone comes with potential risks and side effects. Common side effects include cramping, bleeding, nausea, vomiting, diarrhea, and fatigue.

These are typically mild and similar to the symptoms of a miscarriage, as the body expels the pregnancy tissue. However, in some cases, more severe side effects can occur.

Serious risks associated with mifepristone use include:

**Heavy Bleeding:** While bleeding is expected, excessive bleeding can occur in rare cases, requiring medical attention or even surgical intervention.

**Incomplete Abortion:** In some cases, the abortion may not be complete, leading to the need for a follow-up surgical procedure.

**Infection:** Though rare, infections can occur after the use of mifepristone, especially if any pregnancy tissue remains in the uterus.

Patients should always have access to medical care throughout the process and be aware of signs that may indicate complications, such as extreme pain, heavy bleeding, or fever.

## Contraindications

Mifepristone is not suitable for everyone. Certain medical conditions or circumstances may make its use unsafe, and it is essential to consider the following contraindications:

**Ectopic Pregnancy:** Mifepristone is not effective for terminating ectopic pregnancies, where the embryo implants outside the uterus, often in the fallopian tubes. An ectopic pregnancy requires immediate medical attention and different treatment.

**Chronic Adrenal Failure:** Because mifepristone blocks the effects of progesterone, it can interfere with adrenal function, making it dangerous for individuals with conditions like chronic adrenal failure.

**Allergies to the Medication:** Anyone with known allergies to mifepristone or any of its components should not take the drug.

**Blood Clotting Disorders:** Individuals with blood clotting disorders or on anticoagulant therapy may be at higher risk of severe bleeding after taking mifepristone.

**Long-term Corticosteroid Therapy:** Since mifepristone affects cortisol levels, it should not be used by people undergoing long-term corticosteroid therapy.

# Section 3: The Procedure

Undergoing a medical abortion with mifepristone and misoprostol involves a specific process that must be followed carefully for the procedure to be effective and safe. In this section, we'll walk through how to take mifepristone, what to expect during the procedure, and the possible complications that may arise.

## How to Take Mifepristone

Mifepristone is usually administered in a healthcare setting but can also be taken at home under the guidance of a healthcare provider. The typical regimen involves two steps:

**Taking Mifepristone (First Dose):**

The process begins with taking a single 200 mg tablet of mifepristone orally. This medication works by blocking progesterone, a hormone necessary for maintaining the pregnancy. Without progesterone, the uterine lining breaks down, and the pregnancy is no longer viable.

After taking mifepristone, the patient may go home and wait for the second part of the procedure. It is common to feel little to no immediate symptoms after taking the first dose, though some may experience light bleeding or cramping.

**Taking Misoprostol (Second Dose):**

24 to 48 hours after taking mifepristone, the second medication, misoprostol, is taken.

This can be administered orally (placed in the cheek to dissolve) or vaginally, depending on the medical provider's recommendation.

Misoprostol causes the uterus to contract, expelling the pregnancy tissue. This part of the procedure often induces cramping and bleeding, which can be intense.

It is crucial to follow your healthcare provider's instructions precisely to ensure the effectiveness of the procedure.

## What to Expect During the Procedure

The experience during a medical abortion can vary from person to person, but here are some general things to expect:

**Cramping and Bleeding:** After taking misoprostol, cramping and bleeding typically begin within a few hours. The intensity of the cramps can range from mild to severe, similar to or stronger than menstrual cramps. Bleeding will likely be heavier than a regular period and may include large clots as the body expels the pregnancy tissue. This process usually takes 4 to 6 hours but can vary.

**Additional Symptoms:** Along with cramping and bleeding, you may experience other symptoms such as nausea, vomiting, diarrhea, headache, or chills. These are common side effects of misoprostol and should subside within a day or two.

**Completion of the Procedure:** For most people, the pregnancy tissue will be expelled within 24 hours after taking misoprostol. After the initial heavy bleeding, it is normal to have light bleeding or spotting for up to two weeks. A follow-up appointment is usually scheduled to ensure the abortion is complete, either through an ultrasound or a blood test.

**Emotional Reactions:** Emotional responses can vary widely, and it's important to seek support if needed, whether from loved ones, a counselor, or a healthcare provider. Some people feel relief, while others may experience sadness, anxiety, or mixed emotions.

## Possible Complications

While medical abortion is generally safe and effective, complications can occur, and it is essential to be aware of them. These complications are rare but may include:

**Incomplete Abortion:** In some cases, the abortion may not be complete, meaning that not all pregnancy tissue is expelled. This could result in continued bleeding or the need for a follow-up surgical procedure, such as a dilation and curettage (D&C).

**Heavy Bleeding:** While bleeding is normal, heavy bleeding that soaks through two or more pads per hour for two consecutive hours is a sign of a problem and requires immediate medical attention. Excessive bleeding can lead to anemia or other complications.

**Infection:** Though rare, infections can develop if any tissue remains in the uterus or due to the introduction of bacteria. Symptoms of infection include fever, chills, and a foul-smelling discharge. Prompt medical treatment is necessary if an infection is suspected.

**Severe Pain:** Intense cramping and pain are common, but if the pain becomes unbearable or persists longer than expected, it may indicate a complication such as an incomplete abortion or infection.

**Allergic Reaction:** In rare cases, some individuals may have an allergic reaction to the medications. Signs of an allergic reaction include hives, difficulty breathing, or swelling of the face, lips, or tongue. If these symptoms occur, seek emergency medical attention.

# Section 4: Aftercare

After undergoing a medical abortion, proper aftercare is essential to ensure recovery and prevent complications. This section covers the key aspects of aftercare, including monitoring symptoms, follow-up care, and the disposal of any unused medication.

## Monitoring Symptoms

During the days following a medical abortion, it's important to monitor your symptoms closely to ensure that your body is recovering properly. Here's what to watch for:

**Bleeding:** It is normal to experience bleeding for up to two weeks after the procedure. Initially, this bleeding may be heavy, resembling a heavy period, but it should gradually lighten. If the bleeding becomes excessively heavy (soaking through two or more pads per hour for two consecutive hours) or continues for an extended period, contact your healthcare provider immediately.

**Cramping:** Cramping typically continues for a few days following the procedure. Over-the-counter pain relievers like ibuprofen can help alleviate discomfort. If the cramping becomes severe or does not improve over time, seek medical advice.

**Signs of Infection:** Be aware of symptoms that might indicate an infection, such as a fever above 100.4°F (38°C), chills, foul-smelling discharge, or severe abdominal pain. If any of these occur, it's crucial to seek medical attention promptly.

**General Recovery:** Fatigue and mild nausea may persist for a few days after the procedure. It's important to rest, stay hydrated, and nourish your body as it recovers. Most people feel back to normal within a week or so, but recovery times can vary.

## Follow-up Care

A follow-up appointment is a vital part of aftercare to ensure the procedure was successful and to address any potential complications. This appointment typically takes place one to two weeks after the abortion and may involve:

**Ultrasound or Blood Test:** Your healthcare provider may perform an ultrasound to confirm that the uterus has been completely cleared of pregnancy tissue. Alternatively, a blood test may be done to check for decreasing levels of the pregnancy hormone (hCG), which indicates that the abortion was successful.

**Discussing Symptoms:** Your provider will likely ask about your symptoms, including bleeding, cramping, and any emotional or physical side effects. Be open about your experience so that your provider can offer the appropriate support and guidance.

**Contraceptive Planning:** If you wish to prevent future pregnancies, your provider may discuss birth control options with you during the follow-up visit. Fertility can return quickly after a medical abortion, so it's essential to have a plan in place if contraception is desired.

**Emotional Support:** Recovery isn't just physical—emotional well-being is also important. If you're struggling with feelings of sadness, guilt, or anxiety, don't hesitate to seek counseling or talk to a trusted friend or family member. Your healthcare provider can also refer you to mental health resources if needed.

## Disposal of Unused Medication

If you have any unused mifepristone or misoprostol, proper disposal is important to ensure safety and prevent unintended use. Here's what to do:

**Do Not Flush:** Medications should never be flushed down the toilet, as this can contaminate water supplies and harm the environment.

**Return to a Pharmacy or Clinic:** Many pharmacies and healthcare providers offer take-back programs where you can safely return unused medications for proper disposal. Contact your local pharmacy or clinic to inquire about these services.

**Dispose of at Home:** If a take-back program isn't available, you can dispose of the medication at home. Remove the pills from their original packaging and mix them with an undesirable substance, such as coffee grounds or cat litter. Place the mixture in a sealed plastic bag or container and throw it in the household trash. Be sure to remove or obscure any personal information on the medication packaging before disposing of it.

# Section 5: Mifepristone and Cytotec

Mifepristone and Cytotec (misoprostol) are commonly used together in medical abortions because their combination significantly increases the procedure's effectiveness. In this section, we'll cover how these medications work in tandem, the proper dosage and timing, and how their combined use enhances the success rate of medical abortions.

## Combination Use

The combination of mifepristone and Cytotec (misoprostol) is the standard protocol for medical abortions. Mifepristone initiates the process by blocking the hormone progesterone, which is necessary for sustaining a pregnancy. Without progesterone, the lining of the uterus breaks down, and the pregnancy can no longer be supported.

Misoprostol (Cytotec) is taken after mifepristone to induce uterine contractions, facilitating the expulsion of the pregnancy tissue. The two medications complement each other, making the process more effective than using either medication alone. When used in combination, mifepristone and misoprostol are up to 98% effective in terminating early pregnancies, making this approach the preferred method for medical abortions.

## Dosage and Timing

The effectiveness of the medical abortion regimen relies heavily on the correct dosage and timing of both medications:

**Mifepristone (First Dose):**

The standard dose of mifepristone is 200 mg taken orally in a single dose. This medication is typically administered in a clinical setting, though in some cases, it may be taken at home under medical guidance.

After taking mifepristone, patients are usually advised to wait 24 to 48 hours before proceeding to the next step with misoprostol.

**Misoprostol (Second Dose):**

Misoprostol is typically administered 24 to 48 hours after mifepristone. The standard dose is 800 mcg, which can be taken in one of two ways: orally by placing the pills in the cheek to dissolve (buccal administration), or vaginally.

Misoprostol induces uterine contractions, which help expel the pregnancy tissue. The timing of misoprostol is crucial, as waiting too long or taking it too soon after mifepristone can affect the procedure's success.

Following the correct dosage and timing instructions provided by a healthcare provider is essential for ensuring the effectiveness of the procedure and minimizing the risk of complications.

**Increased Effectiveness**

The combination of mifepristone and misoprostol significantly increases the success rate of medical abortion compared to using either drug alone. Here's how the two medications work together to enhance effectiveness:

**Mifepristone's Role:** Mifepristone prepares the body by stopping the pregnancy from continuing. It cuts off the hormone progesterone, which is necessary for keeping the uterine lining intact. This makes the uterus more receptive to the effects of misoprostol, allowing for a more complete expulsion of the pregnancy tissue.

**Misoprostol's Role:** Misoprostol triggers strong uterine contractions, which help the body expel the pregnancy tissue. These contractions are key to completing the abortion, and the success of the procedure relies on them being powerful and sustained.

**Improved Success Rates:** When used together, mifepristone and misoprostol have an efficacy rate of about 94-98% for pregnancies up to 10 weeks gestation. This makes the combination one of the most reliable methods for medical abortion. Without mifepristone, misoprostol alone is less effective, and there is a higher likelihood of incomplete abortion, requiring additional medical intervention.

In summary, the combination use of mifepristone and misoprostol, with correct dosage and timing, results in a highly effective medical abortion procedure. This method provides a safe, non-invasive alternative to surgical abortion when performed under proper medical supervision.

# Section 6: Frequently Asked Questions

Understanding mifepristone and its role in medical abortion often leads to various questions and concerns. In this section, we'll address some of the most common questions about mifepristone, clarify misconceptions, and provide accurate information to help users feel more informed and confident about the procedure.

Common Questions About Mifepristone

## How long does it take for mifepristone to work?

Mifepristone begins working shortly after it is taken by blocking the hormone progesterone, which is necessary to sustain the pregnancy. However, you may not feel any immediate effects. The process is typically completed when misoprostol is taken 24 to 48 hours later, causing cramping and bleeding as the pregnancy is expelled.

**Is mifepristone safe?**

Yes, when used under the supervision of a healthcare provider, mifepristone is considered safe. Millions of people around the world have successfully used mifepristone for medical abortions. However, like all medications, it has potential risks, and it's important to follow medical advice and attend follow-up appointments.

**Can I get pregnant again after using mifepristone?**

Yes, fertility returns quickly after a medical abortion. You can become pregnant again as soon as you ovulate, which may happen within a few weeks after the procedure. If you want to avoid pregnancy, you should start using contraception as soon as you resume sexual activity.

**How painful is the process?**

Pain levels vary from person to person, but cramping and bleeding after taking misoprostol can be intense, similar to or stronger than menstrual cramps. Over-the-counter pain relief, like ibuprofen, can help manage discomfort. If the pain becomes severe or unmanageable, contact your healthcare provider.

**Will I need to have surgery afterward?**

In most cases, surgery is not required after a medical abortion. The combination of mifepristone and misoprostol is highly effective, but in rare cases, an incomplete abortion may require a surgical procedure, such as dilation and curettage (D&C), to remove any remaining tissue.

Addressing Concerns and Misconceptions

**Is mifepristone the same as the "morning-after pill"?**

No, mifepristone is not the same as emergency contraception (often referred to as the morning-after pill). The morning-after pill, such as Plan B, is used to prevent pregnancy after unprotected sex. Mifepristone, on the other hand, is used to terminate an existing pregnancy.

## Will taking mifepristone cause long-term health problems?

Mifepristone does not typically cause long-term health problems when used for a medical abortion. Most people recover fully without any lasting effects. However, it is important to monitor for any complications and seek follow-up care as advised by your healthcare provider.

## Does mifepristone affect future pregnancies?

Using mifepristone for a medical abortion does not affect your ability to have future pregnancies. It has no known long-term impact on fertility or the health of future pregnancies. However, if you experience any complications, it's important to discuss them with your healthcare provider.

## Can mifepristone cause cancer or other serious diseases?

There is no evidence that mifepristone causes cancer or other serious diseases when used for medical abortion. The medication has been studied extensively and is considered safe for its intended use.

## Is it normal to feel emotional after taking mifepristone?

Yes, emotional responses after a medical abortion are common and vary from person to person. Some people feel relief, while others may experience sadness, guilt, or a range of emotions. It's important to seek support if needed and to talk to a healthcare provider if you feel overwhelmed by your emotions

# BONUS PAGE

## JOURNAL PROMPTS

- **How am I feeling physically and emotionally today after starting the medication? What symptoms am I experiencing, and how am I coping with them?**

..................................................................
..................................................................
..................................................................
..................................................................
..................................................................
..................................................................
..................................................................
..................................................................
..................................................................
..................................................................

- **What thoughts or concerns have been on my mind throughout this process? How have I managed these feelings, and who or what has been supportive for me?**

...........................................................
...........................................................
...........................................................
...........................................................
...........................................................
...........................................................
...........................................................
...........................................................
...........................................................
...........................................................

- **What are my hopes for the outcome of this procedure? How do I envision my life after this experience, and what steps can I take to focus on my well-being?**

...............................................................
...............................................................
...............................................................
...............................................................
...............................................................
...............................................................
...............................................................
...............................................................
...............................................................
...............................................................

• **Describe any changes in my physical symptoms over the past few hours or days. What has surprised me about my body's reaction, and how am I adjusting to it?**

......................................................
......................................................
......................................................
......................................................
......................................................
......................................................
......................................................
......................................................
......................................................
......................................................

- How have I been caring for myself emotionally during this time? What self-care practices are helping me feel more centered and calm?

..............................................................
..............................................................
..............................................................
..............................................................
..............................................................
..............................................................
..............................................................
..............................................................
..............................................................
..............................................................

- **Reflect on any conversations I've had with loved ones or healthcare providers about this experience. How have these interactions affected my feelings about the procedure?**

..................................................................
..................................................................
..................................................................
..................................................................
..................................................................
..................................................................
..................................................................
..................................................................
..................................................................
..................................................................

- **What fears or uncertainties do I still have about the process, and how can I address them in a way that feels safe and supportive?**

...............................................................
...............................................................
...............................................................
...............................................................
...............................................................
...............................................................
...............................................................
...............................................................
...............................................................
...............................................................

- How has this experience shifted my perspective on my body and health? What have I learned about myself through this process?

...................................................
...................................................
...................................................
...................................................
...................................................
...................................................
...................................................
...................................................
...................................................
...................................................

- **What positive affirmations or words of encouragement can I offer myself right now? How can I use these thoughts to stay strong and focused on my recovery?**

..................................................................
..................................................................
..................................................................
..................................................................
..................................................................
..................................................................
..................................................................
..................................................................
..................................................................
..................................................................

- As I move forward, what are my priorities for healing and regaining a sense of normalcy in my life? How can I take small, meaningful steps toward these goals?

..............................................................
..............................................................
..............................................................
..............................................................
..............................................................
..............................................................
..............................................................
..............................................................
..............................................................
..............................................................

Made in United States
Orlando, FL
07 February 2025

58250763R00050